# *Prostate Cancer:*

## Treatment Options for Prostate Cancer

**Joe M. Austin**

# TABLE OF CONTENTS

CANCER

# **INTRODUCTION:**

Prostate malignant growth is a kind of disease that begins in the prostate organ, a pecan-measured organ in men that makes a liquid that helps semen. prostate cancer is the most common cancer among men in the United States.

The prostate organ is situated beneath the bladder and before the rectum. It encompasses the urethra, the cylinder that conveys pee from the bladder out of the body.

Prostate malignant growth typically develops gradually and causes no side effects in the beginning phases. As the disease develops, it can push on the urethra and create some issues with pee, for example, trouble beginning or halting the progression of pee, a need to pee on a more regular basis, or a frail pee stream.

It is also possible for prostate cancer to spread to the liver, bones, and lungs.

## Prostate Cancer

As you get older, your risk of developing prostate cancer goes up. Most prostate malignant growths are analyzed in men beyond 65 years old.

# CHAPTER ONE: DEFINITION

Prostate malignant growth is a sort of disease that begins in the prostate organ, a pecan-measured organ in men. The prostate gland is in front of the rectum and below the bladder. A portion of the fluid that makes up semen is produced by the prostate gland.

Prostate cancer is the most common cancer among men in the United States. Prostate cancer affects approximately one in nine men at some point in their lives.

The stage of the cancer, the patient's age, overall health, and the type of treatment received all influence the prognosis for prostate cancer. Most men with prostate disease are relieved with treatment. Notwithstanding, a few men might encounter repeat malignant growth or difficulties from treatment.

## 1.1. Frequency and Pervasiveness:

The number of new cases of a disease that are diagnosed in a given population over a particular period is known as incidence. Prostate cancer is becoming more common worldwide. In 2020, there were an expected 1,414,250 new instances of prostate malignant growth analyzed around the world. The most noteworthy frequency rates are in North America, Europe, and Australia.

Pervasiveness is the complete number of individuals with sickness in a given populace at a particular moment. Prostate cancer incidence is also rising worldwide. An estimated 14,100,000 men worldwide will have prostate cancer by 2020. Australia, Europe, and North America have the highest prevalence rates.

## 1.2. The Crucial Role of Early Detection:

A type of cancer that grows in men's prostate, a walnut-sized gland that makes seminal fluid, is called prostate cancer.

Prostate Cancer

Prostate cancer detection at an early stage can lead to earlier treatment, which may increase survival chances. There are two primary approaches to early prostate cancer detection: the digital rectal exam (DRE) and the prostate-specific antigen (PSA) test.

The PSA test determines the blood level of PSA. The prostate gland makes a protein called PSA, and an elevated PSA level can indicate cancer. In any case, a raised public service announcement level can likewise be brought about by different circumstances, like harmless prostate growth.

The DRE is a physical exam in which the doctor feels the prostate gland by inserting a gloved finger into the rectum. If the prostate is enlarged or if there are any lumps or irregularities, which could be a sign of cancer, the doctor can feel them.

The American Disease Society prescribes that men converse with their primary care physician about the advantages and dangers of public service announcement testing and DRE beginning at age 50. African American men and men who

# Prostate Cancer

have a family history of the disease may require earlier testing for prostate cancer than other men.

It is frequently possible to treat prostate cancer with surgery, radiation therapy, or hormone therapy if it is discovered early. However, the cancer may have spread to other parts of the body and be more difficult to treat if discovered late.

# CHAPTER TWO: ANATOMY OF THE PROSTATE

In men, the prostate is a gland about the size of a walnut that makes fluid that helps semen. Prostate disease is an illness wherein cells in the prostate develop strangely and can spread to different pieces of the body.

The prostate is situated in front of the rectum and below the bladder. It encompasses the urethra, the cylinder that conveys pee from the bladder to the penis.

The prostate is comprised of three fundamental parts:

The fringe zone: Around the urethra, this is the largest part of the prostate.

The focal zone: The prostate's middle is where this is.

The zone of transition: This is close to the urethra and bladder.

Most of the time, prostate cancer starts in the peripheral zone

## 2.1. Functions Of The Prostate

The production of a fluid that accounts for between 20 and 30 percent of sperm is the prostate's primary function. During ejaculation, this fluid helps to lubricate the urethra and provides sperm cells with nourishment and protection.

assisting with bladder control. During urination, the prostate muscles assist in closing the urethra, preventing urine from returning to the bladder.

releasing hormones that aid in testosterone level control. The prostate believes testosterone into a more intense structure called dihydrotestosterone (DHT). The prostate, penis, and testicles are male sex characteristics that are created and maintained by DHT.

Safeguarding the urethra from disease. The prostate liquid contains chemicals that assist in battling the disease.

## 2.2. Contribution to Male Reproduction:

The prostate is a gland that is the size of a walnut and is located in front of the rectum, below the bladder. About 30% of the semen is made up of this milky fluid. The semen assists with shipping sperm and supports them as they travel through the female contraceptive lot.

The prostate likewise assists with controlling the progression of pee. The prostate contracts when a man is sexually stimulated, assisting in the expulsion of sperm from the penis.

A thin capsule of tissue surrounds the prostate gland. The urethra, the tube that carries urine from the bladder to the penis, can be put under pressure by an enlarged prostate. Having difficulty starting or stopping the flow of urine, having to urinate frequently, or having a weak stream of urine are all signs of this.

Prostate enlargement may also be exacerbated by elevated testosterone levels. Men naturally lose testosterone as they get older, which can help shrink an enlarged prostate.

# CHAPTER THREE: CAUSES AND DEVELOPMENT OF PROSTATE CANCER

Age: Older men are more likely to develop prostate cancer. Prostate cancer risk goes up with age, especially after the age of 50.

The family tree: Prostate cancer is more common in men who have a family history of the disease.

Race: Prostate cancer is more common in African American men than in white men.

Genetics: Prostate cancer risk may be increased by certain gene mutations.

Prostate Cancer

Environment: Prostate cancer risk may be raised by exposure to herbicides and pesticides, among other environmental factors.

Diet: Prostate cancer risk may be increased by eating a diet high in processed foods and red meat.

Obesity: Prostate cancer is increased in people who are obese.

Actual idleness: Prostate cancer is more likely to happen to people who don't exercise.

Although the precise causes of prostate cancer are unknown, it is believed to be caused by a combination of genetic and environmental factors.

When abnormal cell growth begins in the prostate gland, prostate cancer develops. A tumor is formed when these cells divide uncontrollably. The tumor has the potential to grow and spread throughout the body.

## 3.1. Hormonal Impact:

Prostate malignant growth is an illness where cells in the prostate organ develop unusually. Men have a small gland in the shape of a walnut that makes fluid that helps make sperm.

Prostate cancer is influenced by hormones like testosterone in its growth and development. Testosterone is a male sex chemical that is delivered in the balls. It is additionally created in limited quantities by the adrenal organs.

Testosterone can invigorate the development of prostate malignant growth cells. This is because testosterone can tie to receptors on the outer layer of prostate disease cells. At the point when testosterone ties to these receptors, it conveys messages that advise the cells to develop and separate.

Prostate cancer can be influenced by hormones in several ways, including:

Promote the spread of prostate cancer cells to other parts of the body and increase their resistance to treatment by stimulating their growth.

# CHAPTER FOUR: SYMPTOMS AND SIGNS

Prostate cancer typically spreads slowly and may not initially present with symptoms. Be that as it may, as the disease develops, it can cause various issues, including:

Trouble peeing, like a feeble or hindered stream, or the need to pee frequently, particularly around evening time

Excruciating or consuming pee

Blood in the pee or semen

Torment toward the back, hips, or pelvis

Erectile brokenness

Bone agony

Expanding in the legs or feet

Weariness

Weight reduction

Loss of hunger

## 4.1. Symptoms in the advanced stage:

High-level prostate disease is a malignant growth that has spread past the prostate organ to different pieces of the body, like the bones, lymph hubs, or liver.
The extent of the cancer and the organs to which it has spread can have an impact on the symptoms of advanced prostate cancer.

The following are some of the most typical signs of advanced prostate cancer:

Bone ache: This is a typical side effect of cutting-edge prostate malignant growth because the disease cells can spread to the bones. The pain can be mild or severe, and it may get worse as you move around.

Weight reduction: Unexplained weight reduction is one more typical side effect of cutting-edge prostate disease. This is because cancer can make it hard for your body to take in nutrients.

Fatigue: Fatigue, also known as an overwhelming sense of tiredness, is another symptom of advanced prostate cancer. This can make it hard to do ordinary exercises.

Anemia is a low red blood cell count. Anemia is a condition in which there are not enough red blood cells in your body. If the cancer has spread to the bone marrow, where red blood cells are made, this could happen.

Erection problems: The inability to erect or maintain an erection is known as erectile dysfunction. This can occur assuming the malignant growth has spread to the nerves that control erections.

frequent urination, particularly in the evening: This is because the malignant growth can push on the bladder, making it challenging to avoid it.

Prostate Cancer

Urinary discomfort: This can occur assuming the disease has spread to the urethra, the cylinder that conveys pee from the bladder to the beyond the body.

Urine or sperm stained with blood: If the cancer has spread to the prostate or bladder, this could happen.

Inflammation of the legs or feet: This can occur if the disease has spread to the lymph hubs in the legs.

Vermin and nausea: If the cancer has spread to the liver, this may occur.

Weakness: This may occur because the cancer is consuming energy from your body.

Inability to breathe: If the cancer has spread to the lungs, this may occur.

## 4.2. Screening and Analytic Apparatuses:

DRE (digital rectal examination) Through the rectum, a doctor examines the prostate gland. The specialist feels for any knots or anomalies in the organ.

Test for the prostate-specific antigen (PSA): PSA, a protein produced by the prostate gland, is measured by this blood test. A high public service announcement level can be an indication of prostate malignant growth, however, it can likewise be brought about by different circumstances, like an expanded prostate or prostatitis.

Ultrasound of the chest (TRUS): This is an ultrasound test of the prostate organ. To get a better look at the gland, the ultrasound probe is inserted into the rectum.

Prostate biopsy:  A small amount of prostate gland tissue is taken and examined under a microscope during this procedure. The only way to accurately diagnose prostate cancer is through a biopsy.

# CHAPTER FIVE:  STAGES OF PROSTATE CANCER

Staging: It's critical to know how far the cancer has spread after it's been diagnosed. This is called arranging. The following factors are used to determine prostate cancer staging:

Stage A: The malignant growth is bound to the prostate organ.

Stage B: The disease has spread to the original vesicles.

C Stage: The cancer has spread to the prostate-area lymph nodes.

D Stage: The malignant growth has spread to different pieces of the body, like the bones or lungs.

## 5.1. PSA Exam:

The prostate-explicit antigen (public service announcement) test is a blood test that measures the degree of public service announcement in the blood. The prostate gland makes the protein PSA. A high PSA level can indicate prostate cancer, but it can also be caused by conditions like prostatitis or benign prostatic hyperplasia (BPH).

The public service announcement test is not ideal. It can occasionally produce false positive results, which indicate a high PSA level despite the absence of cancer. Additionally, it may occasionally produce false negative results, indicating a normal PSA level despite the presence of cancer.

Beginning at age 50, the PSA test is typically recommended for men. Men with a higher risk of prostate disease, like African American men or men with a family background of prostate malignant growth, might be screened beginning at a prior age.

In addition to the PSA test, other tests are used to screen for prostate cancer. Different tests that might be utilized incorporate the advanced rectal test (DRE) and the prostate biopsy. The DRE is an actual test wherein the specialist embeds a finger into the rectum to feel the prostate organ. The prostate biopsy is a system wherein a little piece of tissue is eliminated from the prostate organ and inspected under a magnifying lens.

The doctor will typically recommend a DRE and a prostate biopsy to confirm the diagnosis of prostate cancer if the PSA test is positive.

## 5.2. Examination of the Digital Rectal (DRE):

A computerized rectal assessment (DRE) is a clinical assessment of the prostate organ through the rectum. For men over 40, it is a common method of screening for prostate cancer.

The DRE is performed by a specialist or other medical services supplier who embeds a gloved, greased-up finger into the rectum. The doctor can then measure the prostate gland's size, shape, and texture by feeling it. A typical prostate organ is smooth and firm. An extended or sporadic prostate organ might be an indication of prostate disease.

The DRE is certainly not an ideal test for prostate disease. It can miss a few malignant growths, and it can likewise prompt bogus up-sides, implying that the test recommends disease when there is none. However, to screen for prostate cancer, the DRE is frequently performed in conjunction with other tests, such as a blood test for prostate-specific antigen (PSA). This is due to the DRE's low cost and ease of use.

The doctor may recommend additional testing, such as a prostate gland biopsy if the DRE results are abnormal. A biopsy is a procedure in which a small amount of prostate gland tissue is taken out and examined under a microscope for signs of cancer.

## 5.3. Biopsy:

A prostate biopsy is a medical procedure in which tiny pieces of tissue are taken from the prostate gland for a microscope examination. It is used to diagnose prostate cancer and assess the disease's severity.

Local anesthesia is usually used for the biopsy, but sometimes general anesthesia is used. A needle is inserted into the prostate gland by the doctor through the rectum. Multiple tissue samples are taken from various parts of the gland.

While the biopsy may occasionally be uncomfortable, it is typically not painful. There is a little gamble of dying, contamination, and injury to the urethra or bladder.

Within a few days, the biopsy results are typically available. Assuming the disease is found, the specialist will examine the treatment choices with you.

There are two principal sorts of prostate biopsy:

Transrectal biopsy: The most prevalent kind of biopsy is this one. The needle is embedded through the rectum and into the prostate organ.

Transperineal biopsy: This biopsy occurs less frequently. Between the scrotum and the anus, the needle is inserted through the skin.

# CHAPTER SIX: TREATMENT

Active monitoring: Men with early-stage prostate cancer who are not likely to spread and do not grow quickly have this option. They undergo routine PSA, biopsies, and imaging tests to keep an eye on them.

Therapeutic radiation: Beams of high energy are used to kill cancer cells in this. It can be used to treat prostate cancer that is localized or to alleviate symptoms of cancer that is advanced.

Chemical treatment: This brings down the degrees of testosterone, which can assist with easing back the development of prostate disease. It is frequently used with other treatments.

Chemotherapy: Drugs are used to kill cancer cells in this. It is in many cases used to treat progressed prostate disease that has spread to different pieces of the body.

Prostate Cancer

Surgery: This eliminates the prostate organ and encompassing tissue. Typically, only localized prostate cancer is treated with it.

Immunotherapy: This is a kind of disease therapy that assists the body's safe framework with battling malignant growth. It works by invigorating the insusceptible framework to perceive and go after disease cells.

Designated treatment: Drugs are used to target specific molecules that are involved in tumor growth and survival in this type of cancer treatment. Prostate cancer that has spread to other parts of the body or returned after treatment can be treated with this type of therapy.

# CHAPTER SEVEN: MANAGING PROSTATE CANCER

Depending on the stage of the cancer, the patient's age, overall health, and preferences, there are numerous ways to manage prostate cancer. Typical ways of overseeing prostate disease include:

Dynamic reconnaissance: This approach is utilized for men with beginning phase prostate malignant growth that isn't developing rapidly. The specialist will intently screen the malignant growth with normal exams and tests. Dynamic reconnaissance isn't a fix, however, it can assist men with staying away from the symptoms of treatment.

Surgery: A medical procedure to eliminate the prostate organ (prostatectomy) is a typical therapy for prostate disease. A radical prostatectomy, which removes the entire prostate gland, and a nerve-sparing prostatectomy, which aims to preserve the nerves that control erections, are two different types of prostatectomy.

Therapeutic radiation: Cancer cells are destroyed by high-energy beams during radiation therapy. Radiation treatment can be utilized to treat prostate malignant growth previously or after a medical procedure, or as an independent therapy.

Chemical treatment: The hormone testosterone, which can help prostate cancer grow, is reduced by hormone therapy. It is possible to use hormone therapy as a standalone treatment or before or after surgery.

Chemotherapy: Drugs are used in chemotherapy to kill cancer cells. Chemotherapy isn't ordinarily used to treat prostate malignant growth, yet it could be utilized in a blend with different medicines.

## 7.1. Results of Treatment:

Radiation treatment: This can cause exhaustion, urinary issues, gut issues, and sexual issues.

Chemical treatment: This can cause hot blazes, erectile brokenness, and deficiency of bone thickness.

Chemotherapy: This can cause sickness, retching, going bald, and weakness.

Surgery: This can cause agony, death, and disease

## 7.2. Care that Helps:

Supportive care is a type of care that helps people with cancer deal with the emotional and practical difficulties of living with cancer as well as the symptoms and side effects of their treatment.

Supportive care for prostate cancer patients can take many forms, including the following:

Prostate Cancer

Management of pain: Prostate cancer often presents with pain, which can be alleviated with a variety of treatments and medications.

Chemical treatment: Prostate cancer tumors can be reduced in size and symptoms can be alleviated with hormone therapy.

Chemotherapy: It very well may be utilized to treat prostate disease that has spread to different pieces of the body.

Therapeutic radiation: It tends to be utilized to treat prostate disease that has not spread to different pieces of the body or to free side effects from cutting-edge malignant growth.

Surgery: Prostate cancer is sometimes treated with surgery. The sort of medical procedure that is done relies upon the phase of the malignant growth and the patient's general well-being.

Nutritional assistance: During cancer treatment, a person's quality of life can be improved by eating well and drinking enough water.

Prostate Cancer



Psychological assistance: Psychological support can help people deal with the emotional challenges of cancer, which can be a very stressful experience.

Palliative consideration: For individuals with serious illnesses, palliative care is specialized medical care. It focuses on alleviating pain and other symptoms and enhancing the patient's and their family's quality of life.

# CHAPTER EIGHT: PROGNOSIS AND SURVIVAL RATES

The stage of prostate cancer, the patient's age, overall health, and the type of treatment they receive all influence the prognosis and survival rates.

Stage: The phase of the malignant still up in the air by how far it has spread. The prognosis for prostate cancer is better than for cancer that has spread to other parts of the body.

Age and general well-being: People who are older and have other health issues typically have a worse outlook than younger people and healthy people.

Treatment method: The sort of treatment that an individual gets can likewise influence their visualization. Prostate cancer treatment options include hormone therapy, radiation therapy, and surgery.

## 8.1. Prognosticating Factors:

The cancer's stage: The extent of a cancer's spread is referred to as its stage. The prognosis for prostate cancer is better than for cancer that has spread to other parts of the body.

Cancer grade: The grade of disease alludes to how strange the malignant growth cells look. Disease with a higher grade is bound to develop and spread than malignant growth with a lower grade.

Public service announcement level: A blood test called the PSA level can determine how much prostate-specific antigen (PSA) is in the blood. The prostate gland makes the protein PSA. A high public service announcement level can be an indication of prostate disease, however, it can likewise be brought about by different circumstances, like harmless prostatic hyperplasia (BPH).

Age: Older men are more likely to develop prostate cancer. Compared to men who are diagnosed with prostate cancer at a later age, younger men typically have a better prognosis.

Race: African American men are bound to foster prostate malignant growth and kick the bucket from it than white men.

The family tree: Prostate cancer is more common in men who have a family history of the disease.

Genetics: Certain quality changes have been connected to an expanded gamble of prostate malignant growth.

Treatment: A man's prognosis can also be influenced by his treatment. Men who get a medical procedure or radiation treatment will quite often have a preferable forecast over men who don't get therapy

## 8.2. Endurance Rates by Stage:

The stage of prostate cancer at the time of diagnosis has a different impact on survival rates.

Prostate Cancer

Stage 1: The malignant growth is small and has not spread to different pieces of the body. Stage 1 prostate cancer has a 5-year survival rate of 96%.

Stage 2: The disease is bigger and may have spread to local tissue. For stage 2 prostate cancer, the 5-year survival rate is 91 percent.

Stage 3: The lymph nodes are now infected with cancer. The 5-year endurance rate for stage 3 prostate malignant growth is 66%.

Stage 4: The malignant growth has spread to different pieces of the body, like the bones or lungs. Stage 4 prostate cancer has a 5-year survival rate of 29%.

# CHAPTER NINE: PREVENTION

You can prevent or lower your risk of prostate cancer by doing the following:

## 9.1. lifestyle changes:

Be healthy in your weight: Being overweight or hefty can expand your gamble of prostate malignant growth. Maintaining a healthy weight through regular exercise and a well-balanced diet is your goal.

Standard active work: By lowering your levels of insulin and insulin-like growth factor (IGF-1), two hormones that have been linked to prostate cancer, exercise can help lower your risk of developing the disease. On most days of the week, aim for at least 30 minutes of moderate exercise.

Prostate Cancer

Eat a nutritious diet: A diet high in fruits, vegetables, and whole grains and low in saturated and processed fats is considered healthy. Antioxidants and other nutrients in these foods may help prevent cell damage, which can help prevent prostate cancer.

Reduce your consumption of red meat: Red meat has been connected to an expanded gamble of prostate malignant growth, particularly when it is handled. Limit your admission of red meat to something like 18 ounces each week.

Give up smoking: Prostate cancer is one of many types of cancer for which smoking is a major risk factor. The best thing you can do to lower your risk is to stop smoking.

Reduce your alcohol consumption: Prostate cancer has been linked to an increased risk of alcohol consumption, particularly in excess. Limit your liquor admission to something like two beverages each day for men.

Take HPV vaccinations: Prostate cancer can be brought on by the human papillomavirus (HPV). Receiving any available immunization shots against HPV can help safeguard against these sorts of diseases.

## 9.2. Dietary Contemplations:

Limit red and handled meats: These meats contain elevated degrees of soaked fat, which has been connected to an expanded gamble of prostate malignant growth. A weekly intake of no more than 18 ounces of red meat and 6 ounces of processed meat is recommended by the American Cancer Society.

Increment your admission of foods grown from the ground: Antioxidants found in fruits and vegetables can help shield cells from damage. At least five servings of fruits and vegetables should be consumed each day, according to the American Cancer Society.

Eat entire grains rather than refined grains: Entire grains are a decent wellspring of fiber, which can assist with lessening irritation. The American Disease Society suggests eating somewhere around three servings of entire grains each day.

Select wholesome fats: Olive oil, nuts, and seeds, all of which contain healthy fats, can help prevent prostate cancer. The

American Malignant Growth Society suggests getting the vast majority of your fat from sound sources.

Drink a lot of water: Prostate cancer risk may also be reduced by staying hydrated, which is important for overall health. Eight glasses of water should be consumed daily, according to the National Cancer Institute.

Drinks with sugar: Sweet beverages are high in calories and can add to weight gain, which is a gamble factor for prostate disease. The American Disease Society prescribes restricting sweet beverages to something like four every week.

## 9.3. Recommendations for Screening:

Age: The American Malignant Growth Society (ACS) suggests that men start talking about the upsides and downsides of prostate disease screening with their primary care physician at age 50. Men who are more likely to develop prostate cancer, such as those who have a family history of the disease, may want to begin screening earlier.

Prostate Cancer

Race: African American men are more likely than white men to develop prostate cancer and die from it. African American men should begin screening at age 45, according to the ACS.

His or her history: Men who have had prostate malignant growth or have had their prostate eliminated are not at an expanded chance of creating prostate disease once more. Thus, they needn't bother with being screened

# CONCLUSION

Prostate cancer is a common cancer that affects men, but it can often be treated, particularly if caught early. There are many gambling factors for prostate disease, including age, family ancestry, and race. Nonetheless, most men who foster prostate disease have no recognizable gambling factors.

Erectile dysfunction, pelvic or back pain, and difficulty urinating are all possible symptoms of prostate cancer. On the off chance that you experience any of these side effects, it is critical to see a specialist immediately.

There is a wide range of tests that can be utilized to analyze prostate disease, including a computerized rectal test (DRE), a prostate-explicit antigen (public service announcement) test, and a biopsy. Your particular circumstances will determine the most appropriate test for you.

The stage of prostate cancer and the patient's overall health determine the course of treatment. Surgery, radiation therapy, hormone therapy, or a combination of these treatments are all options for treatment.

The viewpoint for men with prostate disease is great, particularly assuming the malignant growth is gotten early. Over 99% of men with local
zed prostate cancer survives for five years.

If you have been diagnosed with prostate cancer, it is essential to maintain a positive attitude and collaborate closely with your physician to devise a personalized treatment strategy. You can find a lot of resources to help you deal with prostate cancer, so don't be afraid to ask for help when you need it.